WEIGHT LOSS

The Ultimate guide to achieving your dream body and living a healthier life

Lorraine Bond

TABLE OF CONTENTS

INTRODUCTION

With obesity rates continuously on the rise and its negative impact on overall health and well-being, weight loss has become a major concern for many individuals. While the desire to lose weight may stem from aesthetic reasons, it is important to recognize the numerous benefits that come with shedding excess pounds, such as reduced risk of chronic diseases, improved self-confidence, and increased energy levels. In this book, we will explore various methods of weight loss and their effectiveness, as well as strategies for maintaining a healthy weight long-term. By understanding the importance of weight loss and taking the right approach, we can achieve not only a slimmer physique but also a healthier and happier life.

Why Losing Weight is Important

While fad diets and quick weight loss schemes may promise rapid results, the reality is that sustainable weight loss is crucial for improving overall health and well-being. In this book, we will explore the numerous reasons why losing weight is important.

1. Reduce the Risk of Chronic Diseases:
Being overweight or obese significantly increases the risk of developing chronic diseases such as type 2 diabetes, heart disease, and certain types of cancer.
These health conditions can negatively impact the quality of life and even lead to premature death. Losing weight can reduce the risk of these diseases and lead to a healthier, more fulfilling life.

2. Improve Heart Health:
Carrying excess weight puts a strain on the heart, which can lead to high blood pressure and an increased risk of heart disease and stroke. Studies have shown that losing just 5 to 10 percent of body weight can improve heart health, lower blood pressure, and reduce the risk of cardiovascular disease.

3. Increased Energy Levels:
Being overweight or obese can make everyday tasks feel more challenging and exhausting. This is because carrying excess weight requires more energy, which can lead to feelings of fatigue and lethargy. Losing weight can increase energy levels and make daily activities feel easier and more enjoyable.

4. Improved Mood and Mental Health:
Obesity has been linked to an increased risk of mental health issues such as depression and anxiety. Losing excess weight can improve self-esteem and body image, leading to a more positive outlook on life. Physical activity and a healthy diet also release endorphins, which can improve mood and reduce stress levels.

5. Better Sleep Quality:
Carrying excess weight can lead to sleep apnea, a condition in which breathing stops and starts during sleep, leading to poor quality sleep. Losing weight can improve sleep quality, reducing the risk of sleep apnea, and improving overall health and well-being.

6. Improve Fertility:

Being overweight or obese can affect hormone levels and disrupt the reproductive system, leading to fertility issues in both men and women. Losing weight can improve hormone balance and increase the chances of conceiving.

7. Reduce Joint Pain:
Excess weight puts added pressure on joints, especially in the knees, hips, and back. This can lead to joint pain and increase the risk of conditions such as osteoarthritis. Losing weight can reduce the strain on joints, leading to decreased joint pain and improved mobility.

8. Decrease Medication Dependency:
Being overweight or obese increases the risk of developing health conditions that require medication to manage. By losing weight and

improving overall health, individuals may be able to reduce or even eliminate their dependency on medications.

9. Boost Immune System:
Obesity has been linked to an impaired immune system, making individuals more susceptible to illnesses and infections. Losing weight, together with a healthy diet and regular exercise, can strengthen the immune system and reduce the risk of infections and diseases.

10. Set a Good Example for Others:
Family and loved ones often look to their peers for inspiration and guidance on living a healthy lifestyle. By taking the steps to lose weight and live a healthier life, individuals can serve as role models for

their loved ones and inspire others to make positive changes in their own lives.

Common Obstacles to Weight Loss

1. Lack of discipline: Many people struggle to stick to a consistent diet and exercise routine, making it difficult to lose weight.

2. Emotional eating: Some individuals turn to food as a coping mechanism for stress, boredom or other emotions, which can hinder weight loss efforts.

3. Unrealistic expectations: Setting unattainable goals or expecting quick results can lead to disappointment and frustration, making it harder to stay motivated.

4. Yo-yo dieting: Constantly starting and stopping different diets can be counterproductive and may lead to weight gain in the long-term.

5. Sedentary lifestyle: Lack of physical activity and spending most of the day sitting can make it harder to lose weight.

6. Social pressure and temptation: Social events, holidays, and peer pressure can make it challenging to stick to a healthy diet and exercise routine.

7. Medical conditions: Certain health conditions, such as thyroid disorders or polycystic ovary syndrome, can make it harder to lose weight.

8. Lack of knowledge: Not having a good understanding of proper nutrition and exercise methods can hinder weight loss progress.

9. Financial constraints: Eating healthy or joining a gym can be costly, making it difficult for some individuals to maintain a healthy lifestyle.

10. Plateauing: After initial weight loss, many people hit a plateau where they stop seeing progress, which can be frustrating and demotivating.

11. Lack of support: Trying to lose weight without the support of friends and family can make it more challenging.

12. Negative body image: Negative thoughts and feelings about one's body can lead to self-sabotage and difficulty in achieving weight loss goals.

13. Binge eating: Uncontrollable urges to overeat can lead to weight gain and difficulty maintaining a healthy diet.

14. Hormonal changes: Hormonal imbalances, such as menopause or pregnancy, can make it harder to lose weight.

15. Medication side effects: Some medications, such as antidepressants or corticosteroids, can make it harder to lose weight or lead to weight gain.

Chapter 1: Understanding Weight Loss

A.   The Science of Weight Loss:

Weight loss is a process that involves both the body and the mind. While many focus solely on the physical aspects of weight loss, such as diet and exercise, it is important to understand the science behind why our bodies gain and lose weight.

1. Calories and Metabolism:

The key to weight loss is understanding the concept of calories and metabolism. A calorie is a unit of energy that our bodies use for daily activities and functions. When we consume more calories than we burn, our bodies store this excess energy as fat, leading to weight gain. On the other hand, when we burn more calories than we consume, our bodies use stored fat as energy, resulting in weight loss. Our metabolism, or the rate at which our bodies burn calories, also plays a crucial role in weight loss. Some people have a faster metabolism, meaning their bodies burn more calories at rest. This can make it easier for them to lose weight, while those with a slower metabolism may struggle to shed pounds. However, it is important to note that a person's metabolism can be influenced by various factors, such as genetics, muscle mass, and hormone levels.

2. The Role of Exercise:
Physical activity and exercise play a vital role in weight loss. When we engage in physical activity, our bodies burn more calories, helping us create a calorie deficit

and lose weight. Regular exercise also helps to build and maintain muscle mass, which can increase metabolism and aid in weight loss. Moreover, exercise can have numerous other benefits that contribute to weight loss. It can improve heart health, increase energy levels, and reduce stress and anxiety, among others. It is recommended to engage in at least 150 minutes of moderate-intensity exercise per week for overall health and weight management.

3. Hormones and Weight:
Hormones play a crucial role in regulating our appetite, metabolism, and storage of fat. When hormonal imbalances occur, it can lead to weight gain and difficulty losing weight. One of the most well-known hormones involved in weight regulation is insulin. It is responsible for regulating

blood sugar levels and promoting fat storage. Higher levels of insulin can lead to increased fat storage and weight gain. Other hormones, such as leptin and ghrelin, also play a role in weight loss. Leptin is known as the "satiety hormone" because it signals to our brains when we are full and should stop eating. Ghrelin, on the other hand, is known as the "hunger hormone," and it stimulates our appetite. Imbalances in these hormones can lead to overeating and difficulty losing weight. Certain lifestyle factors, such as lack of sleep and chronic stress, can also disrupt hormone levels and contribute to weight gain. It is crucial to maintain a healthy lifestyle and manage stress to keep hormones in balance and support weight loss.

B.   Different Types of Weight Loss

Weight loss is a hot topic in today's society, with many people constantly searching for the most effective and efficient ways to shed pounds. The truth is, there are many different types of weight loss methods, and what works for one person may not work for another.

Crash Diets vs. Sustainable Lifestyle Changes:

Crash diets, also known as fad diets, are a popular method for quick weight loss. These diets typically involve severely restricting calories or completely eliminating certain food groups, such as carbohydrates or fats. Some examples of crash diets include the cabbage soup diet, the 3-day military diet, and the lemon detox diet. While these diets may result in rapid weight loss, they are not sustainable long-term and can have negative effects on our health. Severely restricting calories can lead to nutrient deficiencies, fatigue, and a slowed metabolism, making it even harder to maintain weight loss in the long run. Additionally, eliminating entire food groups can lead to cravings and an unhealthy relationship with food. On the other hand, making sustainable lifestyle changes is a more effective approach to long-term weight loss. This involves gradually making changes to our diet and exercise habits, rather than drastically cutting calories or eliminating entire food groups. It also focuses on creating a healthy, balanced diet and incorporating regular physical activity as part of our daily routine. While this method may not result in rapid weight loss, it is more likely to lead to long-term success and overall improved health and well-being.

C. Popular Weight Loss Programs Comparison

There is no shortage of weight loss programs on the market, each claiming to be the most effective and scientifically-proven method for shedding pounds. Some popular programs include Weight Watchers, Atkins, South Beach Diet, and Jenny Craig. While these programs may have varying approaches and emphasize different foods or nutrients, the underlying principle is the same – creating a calorie deficit. This means consuming fewer calories than our body needs to maintain weight, resulting in weight loss. However, it's important to note that not all weight loss programs are created equal and what works for one person may not work for another. It's important to do research and consult with a healthcare professional before starting any weight loss program to ensure it is safe and suitable for our individual needs and goals.

D.   Weight Loss Supplements – Are They Worth It?

Weight loss supplements are a multi-billion dollar industry, promising quick and easy weight loss without the need for exercise or dietary changes. These supplements often contain ingredients such as caffeine, green tea extract, or garcinia cambogia, which are believed to aid in weight loss. However, the effectiveness and safety of these supplements are often debated, and many of these products are not regulated by the FDA. While some may provide temporary weight loss results, they may also come with potential side effects and long-term consequences. It's important to remember that there is no magic pill for weight loss and that supplements should not be relied on as the sole method for achieving weight loss goals. As always, consulting with a healthcare professional is recommended before starting any new supplement regimen.

Chapter 2: Setting Your Goals

A. Defining a Healthy Body Weight:

Defining a healthy body weight is an important first step in setting your weight loss goals. It's important to remember that every body is different, and there is no one-size-fits-all approach to determining a healthy weight. There are several methods you can use to determine your healthy body weight:

1. Body Mass Index (BMI): BMI is a measurement of body fat based on height and weight. It provides a general guideline of whether you are underweight, normal weight, overweight, or obese. You can easily calculate your BMI by dividing your weight

(in kilograms) by your height squared (in meters). A BMI between 18.5-24.9 is considered healthy, while a BMI of 25-29.9 is considered overweight and a BMI of 30 or higher is considered obese.

2. Waist-to-Hip Ratio (WHR): WHR is a measurement of the ratio between your waist and hip circumference. It can indicate the distribution of body fat and the health risks associated with it. To measure your WHR, divide your waist circumference (measured at the smallest point above your belly button) by your hip circumference (measured at the widest part of your hips). For women, a WHR of 0.80 or lower is considered healthy, and for men, a WHR of 0.90 or lower is considered healthy.

3. Body Fat Percentage: Unlike BMI and WHR, body fat percentage measures the amount of fat in your body relative to your total body weight. A healthy body fat percentage varies based on age, gender, and activity level. For women, a healthy body fat percentage is generally between 21-33%, and for men, it is between 8-21%.

4. Consulting with a Healthcare Professional: It's always a good idea to consult with a healthcare professional, such as a doctor or registered dietitian, to determine a healthy body weight for you. They can take into account factors like your age, height, weight, and medical history to provide an accurate assessment. Remember, these measurements are just guidelines, and it's essential to focus on overall health rather than just a number on

the scale. Your healthy body weight may be different from someone else's, and that's okay.

B.   SMART Goal Setting:

Once you have determined your healthy body weight, the next step is to set SMART goals that will help you achieve it. SMART stands for specific, measurable, achievable, relevant, and time-bound. Here's how you can apply this to your weight loss goals:

1. Specific: Be specific about what you want to achieve. Instead of saying "I want to lose weight," specify how much weight you want to lose and why.

2. Measurable: Set goals that you can track and measure. This will help you stay motivated and make adjustments if needed.

For example, if your goal is to lose 10 pounds, you can track your progress by weighing yourself once a week.

3. Achievable: Your goals should be challenging but achievable. Set realistic expectations that you can work towards. Losing 1-2 pounds per week is considered a healthy and achievable rate of weight loss.

4. Relevant: Make sure your goals are relevant to your overall health and well-being. Your goal shouldn't only be about losing weight but also about improving your overall health and quality of life.

5. Time-bound: Set a timeline for achieving your goals. This will give you a sense of urgency and a clear deadline to work towards.

C. **Tracking Progress and Celebrating Milestones:**

Tracking your progress is crucial in achieving your weight loss goals. It helps you stay accountable and motivated. Here are some tips for tracking your progress:

1. Keep a food diary: Keeping track of what you eat can help you identify any unhealthy eating patterns and make necessary changes.

2. Use a fitness tracker: A fitness tracker can help you track your daily physical activity and monitor your progress over time.

3. Take progress photos: Seeing physical changes in your body can be motivating.

Taking progress photos every few weeks can help you see how far you've come.

4. Celebrate milestones: Celebrating milestones along your weight loss journey can keep you motivated and on track. Treat yourself to a non-food reward, such as a new outfit or a massage, when you reach a certain goal. Always Remember that weight loss is a journey, and it's essential to focus on progress, not perfection.

Chapter 3: Nutrition for Weight Loss

A.   Understanding Macronutrients

Weight loss is a common goal for many people, but it can be a challenging journey. Along with regular physical activity, nutrition plays a crucial role in achieving weight loss goals. When it comes to nutrition for weight loss,

understanding macronutrients is essential. Macronutrients are the main nutrients that our bodies need in large quantities to function properly – protein, carbohydrates, and fats. Each of these macronutrients has a different role in our bodies and can affect weight loss in various ways.

1. **Protein:** Protein is essential for weight loss as it helps to build and maintain

muscle mass. Protein also has a high thermic effect, which means that it requires more energy to digest, leading to a higher calorie burn. Including lean sources of protein, such as chicken, fish, eggs, and legumes, in your diet can help you feel fuller for longer, reducing the likelihood of overeating. Aim to consume about 0.8-1g of protein per kilogram of body weight per day.

2. **Carbohydrates:** Carbohydrates are the primary source of energy for the body, making them an essential macronutrient. However, not all carbs are created equal when it comes to weight loss. Highly processed carbohydrates, such as white bread, pasta, and sugary snacks, can cause spikes in blood sugar levels and lead to weight gain. Instead, focus on consuming

complex carbohydrates like whole grains, fruits, and vegetables, which provide sustained energy and are more nutrient-dense.

3. **Fats:** Fats have long been demonized in diets, but they are essential for our bodies to function correctly. Healthy fats, such as monounsaturated and polyunsaturated fats, found in avocado, nuts, and oily fish, can promote heart health and aid weight loss. These fats help to keep us feeling satisfied and can reduce cravings for unhealthy, high-calorie foods. In addition to understanding macronutrients, some other key points to consider for weight loss include:

-Calories: Weight loss ultimately comes down to creating a calorie deficit, which means consuming fewer calories than your body burns. It is essential to track your calorie intake to ensure you are not overeating and sabotaging your weight loss efforts.

- Portion control: Along with calories, portion control is crucial for weight loss. Even when consuming healthy foods, overeating can lead to weight gain. Be mindful of serving sizes and use measuring cups or a food scale if needed.

- Balanced meals: Aim for balanced meals that include a combination of protein, carbohydrates, and healthy fats. This helps to keep your blood sugar levels stable and provides sustained energy for your day.

- Mindful eating: Practicing mindful eating can also aid in weight loss. This involves paying attention to your body's hunger cues, eating slowly, and being present during meals. Understanding macronutrients and their roles in weight loss can help you make informed and healthy food choices. It is important to find a balance that works for your body and your weight loss goals. Consult with a registered dietitian or nutritionist for personalized advice on your nutrition journey. Remember that sustainable weight loss takes time, consistency, and a focus on overall health and well-being.

B. Meal Planning for Weight Loss

As the saying goes, "abs are made in the kitchen," and it's true when it comes to weight loss. While exercising is important for overall health and fitness, what you eat plays a crucial role in achieving weight loss goals. Planning your meals can be a powerful tool for weight loss, helping you reach a calorie deficit, practice portion control, and make healthier food choices. Below are some of the key principles of meal planning for weight loss

1. Creating a Calorie Deficit

The most important aspect of weight loss is creating a calorie deficit, meaning you consume fewer calories than you burn. This deficit forces your body to burn stored fat for energy, resulting in weight loss. To create a calorie deficit, you need to determine your daily energy requirements and reduce your calorie intake by 500-1000 calories per day. You can calculate your daily energy requirements using an online calorie calculator, based on your age, gender, height, weight, and activity level. It's important to note that a calorie deficit of 500-1000 calories per day will result in a weight loss of 1-2 pounds per week, which is considered a healthy and sustainable rate.

2. Portion Control and Mindful Eating
In addition to understanding and reducing your calorie intake, portion control and mindful eating are crucial for weight loss. Even if you're consuming healthy foods, eating too much can sabotage your weight loss efforts. To practice portion control, use smaller plates, and measure your food portions using measuring cups or a food

scale. It's also essential to eat mindfully, paying attention to your body's hunger and fullness cues. Avoid distractions such as watching TV or scrolling through your phone while eating, and take your time to savor each bite. This will help you feel more satisfied and prevent overeating.

3. Healthy and Sustainable Meal Ideas When planning your meals for weight loss, it's important to focus on whole, nutrient-dense foods that will keep you satisfied and provide your body with the necessary nutrients. Aim for a balanced diet that includes lean protein, complex carbohydrates, healthy fats, and plenty of fruits and vegetables. Some healthy meal ideas for weight loss include:

- Breakfast: scrambled eggs with vegetables and whole grain toast, overnight oats with fruit and nuts, or a green smoothie with protein powder.

- Lunch: grilled chicken or tofu with quinoa and roasted vegetables, a turkey and avocado wrap with whole grain tortilla, or a mixed greens salad with grilled salmon and a vinaigrette dressing.

- Dinner: baked fish or shrimp with roasted sweet potatoes and broccoli, stir-fry with tofu or lean beef and a mix of vegetables, or a chickpea and vegetable curry with brown rice.

- Snacks: Greek yogurt with berries and almonds, apple slices with peanut butter, or hummus and veggies.

In addition to these meal ideas, be sure to stay hydrated by drinking plenty of water throughout the day. You can also incorporate healthy snacks and treats in moderation, such as dark chocolate or air-popped popcorn. It's important to find a meal plan that works for you, fits your lifestyle, and includes foods you enjoy.

Chapter 4: Exercise for Weight Loss

A.   Finding Your Exercise Style

Finding an exercise style that you enjoy is crucial for sustainable weight loss. Not everyone enjoys going to the gym or running on a treadmill, and that's okay! The key is to find an activity that you genuinely enjoy and look forward to doing. This will make it easier to stay motivated and consistent with your exercise routine. Here are a few tips to help you find your exercise style:

1. Consider your interests: Start by thinking about activities that you genuinely enjoy. Do you like being outdoors? Do you enjoy dancing? Are you a competitive person? These questions can help guide you towards activities that you will likely enjoy.

2. Try different things: Don't be afraid to try out different forms of exercise to see what you like. You can take a dance class, go for a hike, try out a group fitness class, or even join a sports team. The more options you explore, the more likely you are to find something that you truly enjoy.

3. Make it social: Exercising with friends or joining a group class can make working out more enjoyable. Not only does it provide accountability, but it can also make the experience more fun and social.

4. Consider your fitness level: When choosing an exercise style, make sure to take your fitness level into consideration. If you are a beginner, starting with low-impact activities like walking, swimming, or

yoga may be more suitable. As you build your fitness, you can gradually incorporate more challenging exercises.

B. Building a Balanced Workout Routine

A well-rounded workout routine should include a mix of cardio, strength training, and flexibility exercises. Each type of exercise offers unique benefits and combining them will help you achieve your weight loss goals more effectively. Here are some tips for building a balanced workout routine:

1. Incorporate cardio: Cardio, also known as aerobic exercise, is essential for weight loss as it burns calories and promotes overall heart health. Some popular forms of cardio include running, cycling, dancing, and high-

intensity interval training (HIIT). Aim to do at least 30 minutes of cardio most days of the week.

2. Don't neglect strength training: Strength training is often overlooked in weight loss routines, but it plays a crucial role in building lean muscle mass, boosting metabolism, and improving overall body composition. You can incorporate strength training by using free weights, resistance bands, or by doing bodyweight exercises such as push-ups, squats, and lunges.

3. Don't forget about flexibility: Flexibility exercises such as stretching, yoga, and Pilates can help improve range of motion, reduce muscle soreness, and prevent injuries. Don't skip on these important

exercises, and try to incorporate them a few times a week.

## C.	**Cardio vs. Strength Training**

Both cardio and strength training are essential for weight loss, but they offer different benefits. Cardio exercises will burn more calories during the workout, while strength training will help build muscle mass and increase your metabolism. Here's a breakdown:

1. Cardio exercise: Cardio exercise, as mentioned earlier, is crucial for burning calories and improving heart health. It also helps reduce stress, boost mood, and increase endurance. Aim to do at least 150 minutes of moderate-intensity cardio or 75 minutes of vigorous cardio each week.

2. Strength training: Building muscle through strength training is important for weight loss as muscle burns more calories at rest than fat. Additionally, strength training can help improve bone density, posture, and balance. Try to do at least two to three strength training sessions per week, targeting all major muscle groups.

D. Tips for Staying Motivated and Consistent

1. Find an accountability partner: Having someone to hold you accountable can help you stay motivated and consistent with your workouts. This can be a friend, family member, or even a personal trainer.

2. Set realistic goals: Instead of focusing on a specific number on the scale, set achievable goals such as running a 5K or

being able to lift a certain amount of weight. These goals can help keep you motivated and give you a sense of accomplishment.

3. Keep track of progress: Keeping track of your progress, whether it's through a workout journal or fitness app, can help you see how far you've come and motivate you to keep going.

4. Mix it up: Doing the same workout routine every day can quickly become boring and may lead to loss of motivation. Mix things up by trying new exercises, switching up the order of your routine, or changing the intensity.

5. Celebrate small victories: Celebrate your progress, no matter how small. Every little

achievement counts and can help keep you motivated and on track.

Chapter 5: Mindset and Motivation

A.   Overcoming Mental Barriers to Weight Loss

Weight loss is not just a physical journey, but also a mental one. Often, we sabotage our weight loss goals because of mental barriers that hold us back. These barriers may include fear of failure, low self-esteem, lack of motivation, and negative self-talk. To overcome these mental barriers, it is important to first identify and acknowledge them. Reflect on your past weight loss attempts and try to pinpoint where these barriers have come into play. Once you have identified them, it becomes easier to address them. One effective way to overcome mental barriers is to set realistic and achievable goals. This can help build confidence and motivation as you see yourself making progress towards your goals. Additionally, focus on the reasons why you want to lose weight, whether it be to improve your health, feel more confident, or have more energy. This will help keep you motivated and give you a sense of purpose. It is also important to track your progress and celebrate small victories. This can help you stay motivated and remind you of how far you have come. Surrounding yourself with a positive support system can also be helpful in overcoming mental barriers. Seek out friends, family, or a support group who can provide encouragement and motivation on your weight loss journey.

B. Changing Habits and Mindless Eating

Habits play a major role in our daily lives and can often hinder our weight loss progress. This is especially true for mindless eating, where we eat without paying attention to our hunger cues or the types of food we consume. To change these habits, it is important to become more mindful of our eating patterns. Pay attention to your hunger and satiety cues, and eat slowly to give your body time to recognize when it is full. It can also be helpful to keep a food diary to track what and how much you are eating. Breaking the habit of mindless eating also involves making healthier food choices. Stock your kitchen with nutritious and whole foods, and try to limit the availability of unhealthy snacks. Planning and preparing meals in advance can also help prevent impulsive and unhealthy food choices. Lastly, it is important to address any emotional or stress-related eating habits. Find healthy ways to cope with emotions, such as exercise, meditation, or talking to a friend or therapist. These strategies can help break the cycle of mindless and emotional eating.

C. Positive Self-Talk and Building Confidence

The way we talk to ourselves can greatly impact our confidence and motivation. Negative self-talk can lead to self-doubt and sabotage our weight loss efforts. It is important to replace these negative thoughts with positive affirmations and self-compassion. Start by becoming aware of your inner dialogue and when negative thoughts arise. Challenge these thoughts by asking yourself if they are true or if there is another way to look at the situation. Practice positive self-talk and remind yourself of your strengths and accomplishments. Building confidence also involves setting realistic goals and celebrating small achievements. Focus on progress rather than perfection and give yourself credit for every step taken towards your goals. Surrounding yourself with positive and supportive people can also help boost your confidence and motivation.

D. Surrounding Yourself with a Support System

Weight loss can be challenging, so it is important to have a strong support system in place. This can include friends, family, a weight loss support group, or a health coach. Having people who believe in you and your goals can provide motivation, accountability, and encouragement. It is also important to communicate with your support system about your goals and any challenges you may be facing. They can offer helpful advice, hold you accountable, and provide support when needed. Surrounding yourself with positive and like-minded individuals can also help keep you motivated and focused on your weight loss journey. In addition to a support system, it may also be beneficial to seek professional help from a therapist or counselor. They can assist you in addressing any underlying emotional or psychological barriers to weight loss and provide helpful strategies for overcoming them.

Chapter 6: Dealing with Plateaus and Setbacks

Dealing with Plateaus and Setbacks Weight loss journeys can be full of ups and downs. While it can be exciting and motivating to see progress on the scale, there may also be times when your weight loss seems to have stalled or even gone backwards. This is known as a plateau, and it is a common occurrence in weight loss. Dealing with plateaus and setbacks can be frustrating, but it is important to understand why they happen and how to handle them to stay on track towards your goals.

A. **Why Plateaus Happen**

Plateaus occur when your body adjusts to your new diet and exercise routine, causing your weight loss to slow down or even stop. This can happen for a variety of reasons, including a decrease in muscle mass, changes in hormone levels, or a decrease in metabolism. Additionally, if you have been following the same exercise and eating routine for a long time, your body may adapt and become more efficient, making it harder to continue seeing progress.

B. Strategies for Breaking Through Plateaus

Breaking through a plateau requires some adjustments to your routine. Here are some strategies that can help:

1. Change up your workout routine: If you've been doing the same exercises for a while, your body may have adapted to them. Try incorporating new exercises or increasing the intensity of your workouts to

challenge your body and continue seeing progress.

2. Re-evaluate your calorie intake: As your weight decreases, your body may require fewer calories to maintain its current weight. You may need to recalculate your calorie needs and adjust your intake accordingly.

3. Keep track of your food intake: It's possible that you may be consuming more calories than you realize, which could be hindering your weight loss progress. Keeping a food journal or using a calorie tracking app can help you stay on top of your intake.

4. Incorporate strength training: Building muscle mass can help increase your

metabolism, making it easier to burn calories. Adding strength training to your routine can help break through a plateau and prevent future ones.

5. Increase your water intake: Sometimes, dehydration can be mistaken for hunger, leading to overeating. Drinking more water can help you stay full and prevent overeating.

C. Coping with Setbacks and Avoiding the Yo-Yo Dieting Cycle

Setbacks are a natural part of any weight loss journey. You may have a week where you indulge in unhealthy foods or miss a few workouts due to illness or other obligations. These setbacks can be discouraging, but it's important to not let them completely derail your progress. Here are some tips for coping with setbacks and avoiding the yo-yo dieting cycle:

1. Don't beat yourself up: It's important to have a positive mindset and not let setbacks make you feel guilty or ashamed. Instead, use them as learning experiences and move on.

2. Focus on the bigger picture: Weight loss is not just about the number on the scale. Think about how you feel, your overall health, and the progress you've already made.

3. Get back on track: It's easy to let one setback turn into a series of unhealthy choices. Instead, recommit to your healthy habits and get back on track as soon as possible.

4. Seek support: Having a strong support system can help you stay motivated and on track, even during setbacks. Reach out to friends, family, or a professional for support and accountability.

5. Avoid extreme diets: Yo-yo dieting, or constantly gaining and losing weight, can be harmful to both physical and mental health. Instead, focus on making sustainable lifestyle changes that you can maintain long-term. Dealing with plateaus and setbacks is a normal part of any weight loss journey.

Chapter 7: Maintaining Weight Loss

Weight loss is often a challenging journey that requires a lot of dedication, discipline, and hard work. However, the real challenge comes after the weight loss is achieved - maintaining it for the long term. Many people struggle with maintaining their weight loss and often find themselves reverting back to their old habits and gaining back the weight they lost.

A.   Transitioning from Weight Loss to Maintenance Mode:

One of the most important things to remember while transitioning from weight loss to maintenance mode is to not become complacent. This is a common mistake that many people make, thinking that they have achieved their goal and can now relax. However, this can quickly lead to a relapse and weight gain. Instead, focus on making a permanent lifestyle change rather than a temporary diet. This will ensure that you maintain your weight loss for the long term.

B. Strategies for Maintaining a Healthy Lifestyle:

1. Continue Following a Balanced Diet: While it is tempting to go back to eating your favorite unhealthy foods, it is essential to continue following a balanced diet even after achieving your weight loss goal. This will help you to maintain your weight and also keep your body healthy.

2. Experiment with Healthy Recipes: Eating the same foods repeatedly can become monotonous and may lead to cravings for unhealthy foods. Experiment with new

healthy recipes to keep your meals interesting and satisfying.

3. Practice Portion Control: Even though you may have achieved your weight loss goals, it is crucial to continue practicing portion control. This will ensure that you do not overeat and maintain your weight.

4. Make Exercise a Part of your Routine: Exercise not only helps in maintaining weight loss but also contributes to overall health and well-being. Aim for at least 30 minutes of moderate exercise each day to stay active and fit.

5. Stay Hydrated: Drinking enough water is essential for maintaining a healthy weight. It can help curb hunger and prevent

overeating. Aim for at least 8-10 glasses of water per day.

6. Practice Mindful Eating: Be mindful of what you are eating, and pay attention to your hunger and fullness cues. This will help prevent mindless snacking and overeating.

7. Keep a Food Journal: Keeping a food journal can help you track your eating habits and identify any potential triggers for overeating. This can also help you stay accountable and make healthier choices.

C.   Creating a Sustainable Plan for the Future:

To maintain your weight loss for the long term, it is crucial to create a sustainable plan for the future. This means finding a balance between healthy eating, exercise, and indulging in your favorite treats in moderation. Another critical aspect of sustainability is setting realistic goals and expectations. It is essential to understand that weight loss is a journey and that there may be ups and downs. Having a positive attitude and not giving up during setbacks is key to maintaining weight loss.

Chapter 8: Recipes and Meal Plans

HEALTHY BREAKFAST

1. Avocado Toast with Eggs

Ingredients:

- 2 slices of whole grain bread
- 1 avocado
- 2 eggs
- Salt and Pepper
- Olive oil

Instructions:

1. Toast the bread slices in a toaster.

2. In a small pan, heat 1 teaspoon of olive oil over medium heat.

3. Crack the eggs into the pan and season with salt and pepper. Cook for 2-3 minutes on each side.

4. While the eggs are cooking, mash the avocado in a bowl and season with salt and pepper.

5. Spread the mashed avocado on the toast slices.

6. Once the eggs are cooked, place one on top of each toast slice.

7. Sprinkle some more salt and pepper on top and enjoy.

2. Berry Oatmeal
Ingredients:
- 1/2 cup rolled oats
- 1 cup water
- 1/2 cup mixed berries (fresh or frozen)
- 1 tablespoon honey
- 1 tablespoon chopped almonds

Instructions:

1. In a small pot, bring the rolled oats and water to a boil.

2. Reduce the heat and let the oats simmer for 5 minutes.

3. Add in the berries and honey and let it cook for another 2-3 minutes.

4. Once the oats are soft and the berries are cooked, remove from heat.

5. Serve in a bowl and sprinkle the chopped almonds on top.

3. Greek Yogurt Parfait
Ingredients:
- 1/2 cup plain Greek yogurt
- 1/4 cup granola
- 1/2 cup mixed berries (fresh or frozen)
- 1 tablespoon honey

Instructions:

1. In a glass or jar, layer the Greek yogurt, granola, and berries.

2. Drizzle honey on top.

3. Repeat the layering until all the ingredients are used up.

4. Serve immediately or refrigerate for later.

4. Spinach and Mushroom Frittata

Ingredients:

- 1 tablespoon olive oil
- 1 cup sliced mushrooms
- 1 cup spinach
- 6 eggs
- 1/4 cup milk
- Salt and Pepper
- 1/2 cup shredded cheese

Instructions:

1. Preheat the oven to 375 degrees F (190 degrees C).

2. In a medium-sized skillet, heat the olive oil over medium heat.

3. Add in the mushrooms and cook for 3-4 minutes until slightly softened.

4. Add in the spinach and cook until wilted.

5. In a separate bowl, whisk together the eggs, milk, salt, and pepper.

6. Pour the egg mixture over the vegetables in the skillet.

7. Sprinkle the shredded cheese on top.

8. Bake in the preheated oven for 12-15 minutes until the eggs are set.

9. Let it cool for a few minutes before slicing and serving.

5. Overnight Chia Pudding

Ingredients:

- 1/4 cup chia seeds

- 1 cup almond milk

- 1 teaspoon vanilla extract

- 1 tablespoon honey

- Toppings of your choice (berries, sliced bananas, chopped nuts)

Instructions:

1. In a jar or container with a lid, mix together the chia seeds, almond milk, vanilla extract, and honey.

2. Close the lid and shake well to mix all the ingredients.

3. Refrigerate overnight.

4. In the morning, give it another shake and add your desired toppings before serving.

6. Whole Grain Breakfast Burrito

Ingredients:

- 1 whole grain tortilla
- 1/4 cup black beans
- 2 eggs
- 1/4 cup chopped bell peppers
- 1/4 cup shredded cheese
- Salt and Pepper
- Salsa (optional)

Instructions:

1. In a small pan, scramble the eggs and season with salt and pepper.

2. Warm up the tortilla in a separate pan or in the microwave for 10-15 seconds.

3. To assemble the burrito, place the scrambled eggs, black beans, bell peppers, and shredded cheese on top of the tortilla.

4. Optional: Add a spoonful of salsa for extra flavor.

5. Roll up the burrito and enjoy.

7. Apple Cinnamon Overnight Oats
Ingredients:
- 1/2 cup rolled oats
- 1/2 cup almond milk
- 1/4 cup plain Greek yogurt
- 1/4 cup diced apples
- 1 teaspoon cinnamon
- 1 tablespoon honey
- 1 tablespoon chopped walnuts

Instructions:
1. In a jar or container with a lid, mix together the rolled oats, almond milk, Greek yogurt, diced apples, cinnamon, and honey.
2. Close the lid and refrigerate overnight.
3. In the morning, give it a stir and top with chopped walnuts before serving.

8. Tofu Scramble

Ingredients:

- 1/2 block extra-firm tofu
- 1/4 cup chopped onions
- 1/4 cup chopped bell peppers
- 1/4 cup chopped mushrooms
- 1/4 cup frozen spinach
- 1 teaspoon olive oil
- Salt and Pepper
- Whole grain toast (optional)

Instructions:

1. In a pan, heat the olive oil over medium heat.

2. Add in the chopped onions, bell peppers, and mushrooms. Cook for 5-7 minutes until softened.

3. Crumble the tofu into the pan and add in the frozen spinach.

4. Season with salt and pepper and cook for another 5 minutes.

5. Serve with whole grain toast on the side, if desired.

9. Peanut Butter Banana Smoothie Bowl
Ingredients:
- 1 frozen banana
- 1/4 cup almond milk
- 2 tablespoons peanut butter
- 1/4 cup rolled oats
- Toppings of your choice (sliced bananas, chopped nuts, granola)

Instructions:
1. In a blender, blend together the frozen banana, almond milk, peanut butter, and rolled oats until smooth.
2. Pour the mixture into a bowl.
3. Add your desired toppings before serving.

10. Quinoa Breakfast Bowl
Ingredients:
- 1/2 cup cooked quinoa
- 1/4 cup cottage cheese
- 1/4 cup mixed berries (fresh or frozen)
- 1 tablespoon honey
- 1 tablespoon chopped almonds

Instructions:
1. In a bowl, mix together the cooked quinoa and cottage cheese.
2. Top with mixed berries, honey, and chopped almonds.
3. Serve immediately or refrigerate for later.

LUNCH

1. Quinoa and Roasted Vegetable Salad
Ingredients:
- 1 cup quinoa
- 1 red bell pepper, diced
- 1 zucchini, diced
- 1 yellow onion, diced
- 1 cup cherry tomatoes, halved
- 1/4 cup feta cheese
- 2 tbsp olive oil
- 1 tbsp balsamic vinegar
- Salt and pepper to taste

Instructions:
1. Cook the quinoa according to package instructions and let it cool.
2. Preheat your oven to 375°F (190°C).
3. In a large bowl, toss the diced vegetables with olive oil, salt, and pepper.

4. Spread the vegetables on a baking sheet and roast for 20-25 minutes, until they are tender.

5. In another bowl, mix the cooled quinoa with the roasted vegetables and top with feta cheese.

6. Drizzle with balsamic vinegar and serve.

2. Skinny Chicken Caesar Wrap
Ingredients:
- 4 whole wheat tortillas
- 1 cup cooked and shredded chicken breast
- 1/4 cup low-fat Caesar dressing
- 1/2 cup romaine lettuce, chopped
- 1/4 cup cherry tomatoes, halved
- 1/4 cup Parmesan cheese, shredded

Instructions:
1. Lay out the tortillas and divide the shredded chicken among them.

2. Drizzle each tortilla with Caesar dressing.

3. Top with chopped lettuce, cherry tomatoes, and shredded Parmesan cheese.

4. Roll up the tortillas and secure with toothpicks or wrap in foil.

5. Chill in the refrigerator for at least 30 minutes before serving.

3. Mediterranean Tuna Salad
Ingredients:
- 1 can tuna, drained
- 1/4 cup diced red onion
- 1/2 cup diced cucumber
- 1/4 cup Kalamata olives, halved
- 1/4 cup cherry tomatoes, halved
- 2 tbsp olive oil
- 1 tbsp lemon juice
- Salt and pepper to taste

Instructions:

1. In a medium bowl, mix together the tuna, red onion, cucumber, olives, and tomatoes.
2. Drizzle with olive oil and lemon juice.
3. Season with salt and pepper and mix well.
4. Serve over a bed of mixed greens or in a whole wheat pita.

4. Grilled Chicken and Vegetable Skewers
Ingredients:
- 1 lb chicken breast, cut into cubes
- 1 red bell pepper, cut into chunks
- 1 zucchini, cut into chunks
- 1 yellow onion, cut into chunks
- 1 cup cherry tomatoes
- 2 tbsp olive oil
- 2 tbsp balsamic vinegar
- 1 tsp Italian seasoning
- Salt and pepper to taste

Instructions:
1. Preheat your grill to medium-high heat.
2. In a large bowl, mix together the chicken, vegetables, olive oil, balsamic vinegar, Italian seasoning, salt, and pepper.
3. Thread onto skewers, alternating between chicken and vegetables.
4. Grill for 10-12 minutes, turning occasionally, until chicken is cooked through and vegetables are tender.
5. Serve with whole grain couscous or quinoa for a complete meal.

5. Vegetarian Taco Bowl
Ingredients:
- 1 cup quinoa
- 1 can black beans, drained and rinsed
- 1 red bell pepper, diced
- 1 avocado, diced
- 1/4 cup cilantro, chopped

- 1 lime, juiced
- 1 tsp cumin
- Salt and pepper to taste
- Optional toppings: shredded cheese, salsa, Greek yogurt

Instructions:
1. Cook the quinoa according to package instructions and let it cool.
2. In a large bowl, mix together the cooked quinoa, black beans, red bell pepper, avocado, cilantro, lime juice, cumin, salt, and pepper.
3. Serve in a bowl and top with your choice of optional toppings.

6. Chicken and Vegetable Stir-Fry
Ingredients:
- 1 lb chicken breast, cut into strips
- 2 tbsp vegetable oil

- 2 cloves garlic, minced
- 1 inch ginger, grated
- 1 cup broccoli florets
- 1 cup snap peas
- 1 red bell pepper, sliced
- 1/4 cup low sodium soy sauce
- 2 tbsp honey
- 1 tbsp cornstarch
- Salt and pepper to taste
- Brown rice for serving

Instructions:

1. In a large wok or pan, heat the vegetable oil over medium-high heat.

2. Add the chicken strips and cook until browned and cooked through.

3. Remove the chicken from the pan and set aside.

4. In the same pan, add the garlic and ginger and cook for 1-2 minutes.

5. Add the broccoli, snap peas, and red bell pepper and cook until vegetables are tender, about 5 minutes.

6. In a small bowl, mix together the soy sauce, honey, cornstarch, salt, and pepper.

7. Add the chicken back into the pan and pour the sauce over the top.

8. Cook for an additional 1-2 minutes until the sauce thickens.

9. Serve over brown rice.

7. Greek Yogurt Chicken Salad
Ingredients:
- 1 lb cooked and shredded chicken breast
- 1/2 cup plain Greek yogurt
- 1/4 cup chopped celery
- 1/4 cup chopped red onion
- 1/4 cup chopped grapes
- 1/4 cup chopped walnuts
- 1 tsp Dijon mustard

- Salt and pepper to taste
- Lettuce or whole grain bread for serving

Instructions:

1. In a large bowl, mix together the chicken, Greek yogurt, celery, red onion, grapes, walnuts, Dijon mustard, salt, and pepper.
2. Serve on top of lettuce or in a whole grain wrap or sandwich.

8. Cauliflower Fried Rice

Ingredients:
- 1 head cauliflower, grated
- 1 lb shrimp, peeled and deveined
- 1 tsp sesame oil
- 2 cloves garlic, minced
- 1 inch ginger, grated
- 1 cup frozen peas and carrots
- 1/4 cup low sodium soy sauce
- 1 tsp honey

- 2 eggs, beaten
- Salt and pepper to taste

Instructions:
1. In a large wok or pan, heat the sesame oil over medium-high heat.
2. Add the garlic and ginger and cook for 1-2 minutes.
3. Add the shrimp and cook until pink and cooked through.
4. Push the shrimp to one side of the wok and crack the eggs into the other side.
5. Scramble the eggs and then mix in with the shrimp.
6. Add the grated cauliflower and frozen peas and carrots to the wok and cook for 5-7 minutes, until the cauliflower is cooked and the vegetables are tender.
7. In a small bowl, mix together the soy sauce and honey.

8. Pour the sauce over the cauliflower and stir to combine.

9. Cook for an additional 2-3 minutes until everything is heated through.

10. Serve hot.

9. Turkey and Avocado Wrap

Ingredients:

- 4 whole wheat tortillas
- 1 lb deli sliced turkey breast
- 1 avocado, sliced
- 1 cup baby spinach leaves
- 1/4 cup shredded cheddar cheese
- 1 tbsp Dijon mustard
- Salt and pepper to taste

Instructions:

1. Lay out the tortillas and divide the turkey, avocado, spinach, and cheese among them.

2. Drizzle each tortilla with Dijon mustard.

3. Season with salt and pepper.

4. Roll up the tortillas and secure with toothpicks or wrap in foil.

5. Chill in the refrigerator for at least 30 minutes before serving.

10. Lentil and Vegetable Soup
Ingredients:
- 1 cup dried lentils
- 1 onion, diced
- 2 carrots, diced
- 2 celery stalks, diced
- 2 cloves garlic, minced
- 1 can diced tomatoes
- 4 cups low sodium chicken or vegetable broth
- 1 tsp dried thyme
- Salt and pepper to taste

Instructions:

1. In a large pot, cook the lentils according to package instructions and set aside.

2. In the same pot, sauté the onion, carrots, celery, and garlic over medium heat until they are tender, about 5 minutes.

3. Add the can of diced tomatoes (with the juice) and let it cook for an additional 2-3 minutes.

4. Add the cooked lentils, chicken or vegetable broth, dried thyme, salt, and pepper.

5. Bring to a boil, then reduce the heat and let it simmer for 20-25 minutes.

6. Serve hot.

DINNER RECIPES

1. Baked Lemon Chicken with Roasted Vegetables
Ingredients:
- 4 skinless, boneless chicken breasts
- Juice of 1 lemon
- 2 cloves of garlic, minced
- 1 tsp dried oregano
- 1 tsp dried thyme
- Salt and pepper to taste
- 1 red bell pepper, sliced
- 1 zucchini, sliced
- 1 yellow squash, sliced
- 1 red onion, sliced
- 1 tbsp olive oil

Instructions:
1. Preheat the oven to 375°F.

2. In a small bowl, mix together the lemon juice, minced garlic, oregano, thyme, salt, and pepper.

3. Place the chicken breasts in a baking dish and pour the marinade over them, making sure they are coated evenly.

4. In a separate bowl, toss the sliced vegetables with olive oil, salt, and pepper.

5. Arrange the vegetables around the chicken in the baking dish.

6. Bake for 25-30 minutes, or until the chicken is cooked through and the vegetables are tender.

2. Zucchini Noodle Stir-Fry with Shrimp
Ingredients:
- 2 medium zucchini, spiralized into noodles
- 1 lb shrimp, peeled and deveined
- 1 tbsp olive oil

- 2 cloves of garlic, minced
- 1 tsp grated ginger
- 1 red bell pepper, sliced
- 1 cup snow peas
- 2 tbsp soy sauce
- 1 tsp honey
- 1 tsp sesame oil
- Salt and pepper to taste

Instructions:
1. In a large skillet, heat the olive oil over medium heat.
2. Add the garlic and ginger and sauté for 1 minute.
3. Add the shrimp and cook for 2-3 minutes, until they turn pink.
4. Add the sliced red bell pepper and snow peas and cook for an additional 2-3 minutes.

5. In a small bowl, mix together the soy sauce, honey, and sesame oil.

6. Pour the sauce over the shrimp and vegetables and stir to coat.

7. Add the zucchini noodles to the skillet and cook for 2-3 minutes, until they are tender.

8. Serve hot.

3. Quinoa Veggie Bowl
Ingredients:
- 1 cup quinoa
- 2 cups water
- 1 tbsp olive oil
- 2 cloves of garlic, minced
- 1 red onion, diced
- 1 red bell pepper, diced
- 1 zucchini, diced
- 1 cup cherry tomatoes, halved
- 1 can black beans, drained and rinsed

- 1 avocado, chopped
- 1 lime, juiced
- Salt and pepper to taste

Instructions:
1. In a small saucepan, bring the water to a boil and add the quinoa.
2. Reduce heat to low, cover, and simmer for 15 minutes, until the water is absorbed.
3. In a large skillet, heat the olive oil over medium heat.
4. Add the garlic and sauté for 1 minute.
5. Add the red onion, bell pepper, and zucchini and cook for 5-7 minutes, until tender.
6. Add the cherry tomatoes and black beans to the skillet and cook for an additional 2-3 minutes.
7. In a small bowl, mix together the avocado, lime juice, and salt and pepper.

8. Serve the quinoa topped with the vegetable mixture and avocado.

4. Herb-Crusted Baked Salmon with Roasted Asparagus
Ingredients:
- 4 salmon fillets
- 1 tbsp olive oil
- 1 tsp dried thyme
- 1 tsp dried rosemary
- 1 tsp dried oregano
- Salt and pepper to taste
- 1 lb asparagus, trimmed
- 1 tbsp olive oil
- Salt and pepper to taste
- Lemon wedges for serving

Instructions:
1. Preheat the oven to 375°F.

2. In a small bowl, mix together the olive oil, thyme, rosemary, oregano, salt, and pepper.

3. Place the salmon fillets on a baking dish and spread the herb mixture over them.

4. Bake for 15-20 minutes, until the salmon is cooked through.

5. In a separate baking dish, toss the asparagus with olive oil, salt and pepper.

6. Place the asparagus next to the salmon in the oven for the last 10 minutes of cooking.

7. Serve the salmon and asparagus with lemon wedges.

5. Turkey and Vegetable Stir-Fry with Brown Rice

Ingredients:

- 1 cup brown rice

- 2 cups water

- 1 lb ground turkey

- 1 tbsp olive oil
- 1 tsp grated ginger
- 2 cloves of garlic, minced
- 1 red bell pepper, diced
- 1 zucchini, diced
- 1 cup broccoli florets
- 2 tbsp soy sauce
- Salt and pepper to taste

Instructions:

1. In a small saucepan, bring the water to a boil and add the brown rice.

2. Reduce heat to low, cover, and simmer for 45 minutes.

3. In a large skillet, heat the olive oil over medium heat.

4. Add the ground turkey and cook until browned, breaking it up into small pieces.

5. Add the ginger and garlic and sauté for 1 minute.

6. Add the red bell pepper, zucchini, and broccoli to the skillet and cook for 5-7 minutes, until the vegetables are tender.
7. Stir in the soy sauce and season with salt and pepper to taste.
8. Serve over the cooked brown rice.

6. Grilled Chicken Salad with Balsamic Vinaigrette
Ingredients:
- 4 skinless, boneless chicken breasts
- 1 tbsp olive oil
- Salt and pepper to taste
- 8 cups mixed greens
- 1 cup cherry tomatoes, halved
- 1 avocado, diced
- 1/4 cup sliced red onion
- 1/4 cup crumbled feta cheese
- 1/4 cup balsamic vinegar
- 2 tbsp olive oil

- 1 tsp Dijon mustard
- 1 tsp honey
- Salt and pepper to taste

Instructions:
1. Preheat the grill to medium heat.
2. Brush the chicken breasts with olive oil and season with salt and pepper.
3. Grill the chicken for 6-8 minutes on each side, until cooked through.
4. In a large bowl, toss together the mixed greens, cherry tomatoes, avocado, red onion, and feta cheese.
5. In a small bowl, whisk together the balsamic vinegar, olive oil, mustard, honey, salt, and pepper to make the dressing.
6. Serve the grilled chicken on top of the salad and drizzle with balsamic vinaigrette.

7. Veggie and Tofu Stir-Fry with Brown Rice
Ingredients:
- 1 cup brown rice
- 2 cups water
- 1 block tofu, diced
- 1 tbsp sesame oil
- 1 tbsp soy sauce
- 1 tbsp rice vinegar
- 1 tbsp honey
- 2 cloves of garlic, minced
- 1 tsp grated ginger
- 1 red bell pepper, sliced
- 1 cup snow peas
- 1 cup carrots, sliced
- 1 cup broccoli florets

Instructions:
1. In a small saucepan, bring the water to a boil and add the brown rice.

2. Reduce heat to low, cover, and simmer for 45 minutes.

3. In a large skillet, heat the sesame oil over medium heat.

4. Add the diced tofu and sauté until golden brown.

5. In a small bowl, whisk together the soy sauce, rice vinegar, honey, garlic, and ginger.

6. Pour the sauce over the tofu and continue cooking for 2-3 minutes.

7. Add the sliced red pepper, snow peas, carrots, and broccoli to the skillet.

8. Cook for an additional 5-7 minutes, until the vegetables are tender.

9. Serve over the cooked brown rice.

8. Baked Cod with Lemon Butter and Broccoli

Ingredients:

- 4 cod fillets
- 1 tbsp olive oil
- Salt and pepper to taste
- 2 lemons, sliced
- 4 tbsp butter
- 2 cloves of garlic, minced
- 1 lb broccoli, chopped
- Olive oil cooking spray

Instructions:
1. Preheat the oven to 375°F.
2. Place the cod fillets on a baking sheet and drizzle with olive oil.
3. Season with salt and pepper to taste.
4. Arrange lemon slices on top of each fillet.
5. In a small saucepan, melt the butter and add the minced garlic.
6. Pour the butter mixture over the cod fillets.

7. In a separate baking dish, toss the chopped broccoli in olive oil cooking spray.

8. Bake the cod and broccoli for 12-15 minutes, until the cod is cooked through and the broccoli is tender.

9. Lentil and Vegetable Soup
Ingredients:
- 1 tbsp olive oil
- 1 onion, chopped
- 2 cloves of garlic, minced
- 1 cup carrots, chopped
- 1 cup celery, chopped
- 1 cup green beans, chopped
- 1 can diced tomatoes
- 6 cups vegetable broth
- 1 cup dried lentils
- 1 tsp dried basil
- 1 tsp dried oregano
- Salt and pepper to taste

Instructions:

1. In a large pot, heat the olive oil over medium heat.

2. Add the onion and garlic and sauté until softened.

3. Add the carrots, celery, and green beans to the pot and cook for 5 minutes.

4. Stir in the diced tomatoes and vegetable broth.

5. Add the dried lentils, basil, oregano, salt, and pepper.

6. Bring the soup to a boil, then reduce the heat and let simmer for 30 minutes.

7. Serve hot.

10. Grilled Shrimp and Vegetable Skewers with Quinoa Salad

Ingredients:

- 1 lb shrimp, peeled and deveined

- 1 red bell pepper, cut into chunks
- 1 zucchini, cut into chunks
- 1 red onion, cut into chunks
- 1 cup quinoa
- 2 cups water
- 1/4 cup olive oil
- 2 tbsp balsamic vinegar
- 1 tsp Dijon mustard
- 1 tsp honey
- Salt and pepper to taste

Instructions:

1. In a small saucepan, bring the water to a boil and add the quinoa.

2. Reduce heat to low, cover, and simmer for 15 minutes.

3. In a small bowl, whisk together the olive oil, balsamic vinegar, mustard, honey, salt, and pepper to make the dressing.

4. In a separate bowl, toss the shrimp, red bell pepper, zucchini, and red onion with the dressing.

5. Thread the shrimp and vegetables onto skewers.

6. Heat a grill or grill pan to medium heat and cook the skewers for 5-6 minutes on each side, until the shrimp are pink and the vegetables are tender.

7. Serve with the quinoa salad.

DELICIOUS AND NUTRITIOUS SNACK IDEAS

1. Avocado Toast with Soft Boiled Egg
Ingredients:
- 1 ripe avocado
- 2 slices of whole wheat bread
- 2 eggs

- Salt and pepper to taste
- Optional toppings: cherry tomatoes, feta cheese, chia seeds

Instructions:
1. Cut open the avocado and remove the pit. Scoop out the flesh into a bowl and mash it with a fork until desired consistency.
2. Toast the bread slices until golden brown.
3. In a saucepan, bring water to a boil and carefully add the eggs. Let them cook for 6-7 minutes for a soft boiled egg.
4. Remove the eggs from the hot water and peel them.
5. Spread the mashed avocado on the toasted bread slices and top each with a soft boiled egg.
6. Sprinkle salt and pepper to taste.
7. Add optional toppings for added flavor and nutrition.

8. Serve and enjoy your creamy and protein-packed avocado toast!

2. Berry and Yogurt Parfait
Ingredients:
- 1 cup Greek yogurt
- 1/2 cup mixed berries (strawberries, blueberries, raspberries)
- 1/4 cup granola
- Honey or agave syrup (optional)

Instructions:
1. In a glass or jar, layer 1/4 cup of yogurt, followed by a layer of mixed berries.
2. Repeat layers until all the yogurt and berries are used up.
3. Top with granola for added crunch.
4. Drizzle honey or agave syrup on top, if desired.

5. Serve and enjoy your protein-packed and nutrient-dense parfait as a filling and delicious snack!

3. Energy Bites
Ingredients:
- 1 cup rolled oats
- 1/2 cup peanut butter
- 1/4 cup honey
- 1/4 cup dark chocolate chips
- 1/4 cup shredded coconut
- 1 tsp vanilla extract
- Optional add-ins: chia seeds, flax seeds, dried cranberries, chopped almonds

Instructions:
1. In a mixing bowl, combine rolled oats, peanut butter, honey, shredded coconut, and vanilla extract.

2. Add in any optional add-ins of your choice and mix well.

3. Roll the mixture into small bite-size balls.

4. Place on a baking sheet lined with parchment paper and refrigerate for 30 minutes.

5. Melt dark chocolate chips in the microwave or on the stove.

6. Dip the chilled energy bites in the melted chocolate and place them back on the parchment paper.

7. Return them to the refrigerator for an additional 15 minutes.

8. Serve and enjoy these delicious and nutritious energy bites as a pre or post-workout snack!

4. Caprese Skewers
Ingredients:
- Cherry tomatoes

- Fresh basil leaves
- Mozzarella balls
- Balsamic vinegar
- Olive oil
- Salt and pepper to taste

Instructions:

1. On a skewer, thread a cherry tomato, followed by a basil leaf and a mozzarella ball.

2. Repeat this pattern until the skewer is filled.

3. In a small bowl, mix together balsamic vinegar, olive oil, salt, and pepper to make a vinaigrette.

4. Drizzle the vinaigrette over the skewers before serving.

5. These caprese skewers are perfect for a quick and refreshing snack, and are packed

with antioxidants and healthy fats from the olive oil.

5. Apple Nachos
Ingredients:
- 2 apples
- 1/4 cup creamy peanut butter
- 1/4 cup dark chocolate chips
- 1/4 cup chopped nuts (almonds, walnuts, or pecans)

Instructions:
1. Slice the apples into thin rounds.
2. Arrange them on a plate in a single layer.
3. In a small microwave-safe bowl, melt the peanut butter for 30 seconds.
4. Drizzle the melted peanut butter over the sliced apples.
5. Sprinkle dark chocolate chips and chopped nuts on top.

6. Microwave for an additional 30 seconds or until the chocolate chips are melted.

7. Serve and enjoy your sweet and satisfying apple nachos as a guilt-free snack option!

C. Sample Meal Plans for Different Calorie Intake Levels

Day 1:

1200 Calorie Meal Plan:

Breakfast: Avocado and poached egg on whole grain toast (300 calories)

Lunch: Quinoa and black bean salad with grilled chicken (350 calories)

Dinner: Baked salmon with roasted vegetables (400 calories)

Snack: Small apple with 1 tbsp almond butter (150 calories)

1500 Calorie Meal Plan:

Breakfast: Greek yogurt with berries and almonds (300 calories)

Lunch: Turkey and avocado wrap with whole wheat tortilla (400 calories)

Dinner: Grilled chicken breast with quinoa and steamed broccoli (450 calories)

Snack: Carrots and celery sticks with hummus (150 calories)

2000 Calorie Meal Plan:

Breakfast: Oatmeal with almond milk, banana, and cinnamon (400 calories)

Lunch: Grilled shrimp and vegetable stir-fry with brown rice (600 calories)

Dinner: Baked sweet potato with black bean and corn salsa and grilled chicken (600 calories)

Snack: Yogurt and fruit parfait with granola (400 calories)

Day 2:
1200 Calorie Meal Plan:
Breakfast: Spinach and feta egg white omelette (300 calories)
Lunch: Grilled chicken Caesar salad (350 calories)
Dinner: Turkey and vegetable meatloaf with roasted sweet potatoes (400 calories)
Snack: Small orange with 1 oz almonds (150 calories)

1500 Calorie Meal Plan:
Breakfast: Whole grain toast with avocado and tomato slices (300 calories)
Lunch: Quinoa and vegetable stuffed bell peppers (400 calories)
Dinner: Baked tilapia with roasted asparagus and quinoa (450 calories)
Snack: Air-popped popcorn (150 calories)

2000 Calorie Meal Plan:
Breakfast: Protein smoothie with banana, spinach, and almond milk (400 calories)
Lunch: Black bean and vegetable burrito with side salad (600 calories)
Dinner: Grilled chicken and vegetable kebabs with quinoa (600 calories)
Snack: 1 oz dark chocolate with 1 small apple (400 calories)

Day 3:
1200 Calorie Meal Plan:
Breakfast: Cottage cheese and fruit bowl (300 calories)
Lunch: Whole grain wrap with turkey, avocado, and hummus (350 calories)
Dinner: Vegetable stir-fry with tofu and brown rice (400 calories)
Snack: Baby carrots with 2 tbsp ranch dressing (150 calories)

1500 Calorie Meal Plan:

Breakfast: Whole grain waffles topped with Greek yogurt and fruit (300 calories)

Lunch: Grilled chicken and vegetable kebab on a skewer (450 calories)

Dinner: Baked cod with roasted vegetables and quinoa (450 calories)

Snack: Small apple with 1 oz cheddar cheese (150 calories)

2000 Calorie Meal Plan:

Breakfast: Vegetable and mushroom frittata (400 calories)

Lunch: Whole grain pita with hummus, turkey, and veggies (600 calories)

Dinner: Grilled sirloin steak with roasted sweet potatoes and green beans (600 calories)

Snack: Whole grain crackers with cheese and grapes (400 calories)

Day 4:

1200 Calorie Meal Plan:

Breakfast: Berry and spinach protein shake (300 calories)

Lunch: Grilled chicken and vegetable skewer with quinoa (350 calories)

Dinner: Spaghetti squash with turkey meatballs and marinara sauce (400 calories)

Snack: Small banana with 1 tbsp almond butter (150 calories)

1500 Calorie Meal Plan:

Breakfast: Whole grain English muffin with scrambled eggs and avocado (300 calories)

Lunch: Chickpea and vegetable curry over brown rice (450 calories)

Dinner: Baked pork tenderloin with roasted vegetables and quinoa (450 calories)

Snack: Celery sticks with hummus and 1 oz cashews (150 calories)

2000 Calorie Meal Plan:

Breakfast: Whole grain French toast with berries and Greek yogurt (400 calories)
Lunch: Grilled vegetable and chicken wrap with side salad (600 calories)
Dinner: Baked salmon with quinoa and steamed broccoli (600 calories)
Snack: Whole grain crackers with hummus and cheese (400 calories)

Day 5:
1200 Calorie Meal Plan:

Breakfast: Poached egg on whole grain toast with spinach and tomato slices (300 calories)
Lunch: Quinoa and black bean salad with grilled shrimp (350 calories)

Dinner: Baked chicken breast with roasted Brussels sprouts and sweet potatoes (400 calories)

Snack: Small Greek yogurt with 1/4 cup berries (150 calories)

1500 Calorie Meal Plan:

Breakfast: Whole grain bagel with cream cheese, smoked salmon, and cucumber slices (300 calories)

Lunch: Tuna salad with whole wheat crackers and fruit (450 calories)

Dinner: Grilled vegetable and tofu stir-fry with brown rice (450 calories)

Snack: Small orange with 1 oz almonds (150 calories)

2000 Calorie Meal Plan:

Breakfast: Whole grain toast with scrambled eggs, avocado, and tomato slices (400 calories)

Lunch: Grilled chicken and vegetable panini with side salad (600 calories)

Dinner: Baked tilapia with quinoa and steamed broccoli (600 calories)

Snack: Small apple with 1 oz cheddar cheese (400 calories)

Day 6:
1200 Calorie Meal Plan:

Breakfast: Overnight oats with almond milk, banana, and cinnamon (300 calories)

Lunch: Grilled turkey and vegetable wrap with side salad (350 calories)

Dinner: Baked tofu with roasted vegetables and quinoa (400 calories)

Snack: Carrots and celery sticks with 2 tbsp hummus (150 calories)

1500 Calorie Meal Plan:

Breakfast: Whole grain pancakes with Greek yogurt and fruit (300 calories)

Lunch: Grilled chicken and vegetable skewer with hummus and whole wheat pita (450 calories)

Dinner: Baked cod with quinoa and steamed asparagus (450 calories)

Snack: Small banana with 1 oz cashews (150 calories)

2000 Calorie Meal Plan:

Breakfast: Veggie and cheese omelette with whole grain toast (400 calories)

Lunch: Grilled vegetable and chicken wrap with side salad and fruit (600 calories)

Dinner: Grilled sirloin steak with sweet potato fries and roasted Brussels sprouts (600 calories)
Snack: Air-popped popcorn (400 calories)

Day 7:
1200 Calorie Meal Plan:
Breakfast: Scrambled eggs with spinach and feta cheese (300 calories)
Lunch: Chickpea and vegetable salad with grilled chicken (350 calories)
Dinner: Baked pork tenderloin with roasted sweet potatoes and green beans (400 calories)
Snack: Small apple with 1 tbsp almond butter (150 calories)

1500 Calorie Meal Plan:

Breakfast: Whole grain English muffin with avocado, smoked salmon, and tomato slices (300 calories)

Lunch: Quinoa and black bean salad with grilled shrimp (450 calories)

Dinner: Baked chicken breast with roasted vegetables and quinoa (450 calories)

Snack: Small Greek yogurt with 1/4 cup berries (150 calories)

2000 Calorie Meal Plan:

Breakfast: Veggie and cheese frittata with whole grain toast (400 calories)

Lunch: Turkey and vegetable wrap with hummus and Greek salad (600 calories)

Dinner: Baked salmon with quinoa and steamed broccoli (600 calories)

Snack: Small apple with 1 oz cheddar cheese (400 calories)

Chapter 9: Final Thoughts

A. Celebrating Your Accomplishments:

Losing weight is not an easy task and it requires a lot of determination, hard work and persistence. Therefore, it is important to celebrate your accomplishments, big or small, along the weight loss journey. This can help to keep you motivated and boost your self-confidence. Celebrations can be in the form of treating yourself to a new outfit, getting a new haircut or indulging in your favorite healthy meal. It is important to recognize and acknowledge your efforts and progress.

B. Reflection and Gratitude:

Amidst the hustle and bustle of achieving weight loss goals, it is crucial to take a step back and reflect on your journey. Reflecting on your progress can help you to identify what worked for you and what didn't. This will not only help you in avoiding any mistakes in the future but also give you a sense of accomplishment and pride. It is also important to express gratitude towards yourself for the hard work you have put in and towards the people who supported and encouraged you along the way.

C. Continual Self-Care and Progression:

Maintaining a healthy weight is not a one-time achievement but a continuous process. It is important to continue practicing self-care and maintaining healthy habits even after reaching your desired weight. This can include regular exercise, mindful eating, and self-care activities like getting enough rest, managing stress, and nurturing your mental and emotional well-being. Keep setting new goals and strive for progress rather than perfection. Remember, weight loss is not just about reaching a number on the scale, but about overall health and well-being.

In conclusion, achieving and maintaining a healthy weight is a goal that requires determination, dedication, and consistency. By implementing a balanced and sustainable approach to nutrition, exercise, and self-care, individuals can successfully lose weight and improve their overall health. It is important to remember that weight loss is a journey, not a destination, and setbacks and challenges will inevitably arise. However, with a positive mindset and support from loved ones, the benefits of achieving a healthy weight – including increased energy, confidence, and reduced risk of chronic diseases – make the effort worthwhile. By making informed and mindful choices, anyone can achieve their weight loss goals and live a fulfilling, healthy life.

Good luck in your weight loss journey and see you on the side of victory.